About the Author

Katelyn Owens is a twenty-four-year-old writer and Criminology and Sociology student at The Open University. She has lived in the United States, United Kingdom, Switzerland, and France. By sharing her own experience in addiction and recovery, she hopes to help other addicts and their families cope with and learn more about addiction.

Addiction
By a young adult, for young adults

Katelyn M. Owens

Addiction
By a young adult, for young adults

Olympia Publishers
London

www.olympiapublishers.com

OLYMPIA PAPERBACK EDITION

A CIP catalogue record for this title is
available from the British Library.

ISBN: 978-1-80074-238-3

The opinions expressed in this book are the author's own and do
not reflect the views of the publisher, author's employer,
organization, committee or other group or individual.

First Published in 2022

Olympia Publishers
Tallis House
2 Tallis Street
London
EC4Y 0AB
Printed in Great Britain

Dedication

To all the addicts born today and who lost their lives to addiction today.

Acknowledgements

I would like to give special thanks to several people for helping me throughout my recovery journey and the process of writing, editing, and publishing this book.

First and foremost, thank you to my amazing partner, Chris, who has been there for me since day one. You have given me true, unconditional love in times of hardship. I will be forever grateful for your patience with and belief in me.

Second, thank you, Mom and Dad, for your love and support throughout my tumultuous journey. Your constant support has grounded me throughout my experiences, and I look forward to continuing to rebuild our relationships as time goes on.

Third, a huge thank you to all of my wonderful grandparents. You have been voices of reason throughout my life, including my addiction, and I wouldn't have been able to stay sane without you.

Fourth, thank you to all of my other loved ones for loving me despite my flaws and realizing my true worth. When I first came out about my addiction, I was scared I would be condescended or judged. I couldn't have been more wrong.

Fifth, thank you to my therapist, who has supported me in overcoming my addiction. Your wisdom and experience have touched me and helped inspire this book. Without your guidance, I wouldn't be where I am today.

Last, but not least, thank you to all of the other addicts I have met, who have provided me with an undeniable sense of solidarity throughout my recovery. My continued recovery would not be possible without the bond we share, and I cannot express how grateful I am to have met all of you.

I would also like to give special thanks to everyone who has read my book. Thank you for your interest, attention, and desire to learn more about me and addiction.

Introduction

Addiction affects millions of people worldwide each year. I am one of those people. If you are reading this book, you may be one of those people too. Maybe someone you know is one of those people. While addicts do a good job of isolating from the world, addiction is not an isolated event. Just like chicken pox or the flu, the disease of addiction affects people everywhere regardless of age, sex, gender, race, religion, culture, ethnicity, or socio-economic status.

Although addiction does not discriminate against age, I am writing to young adults in particular, because that is the age at which I realized I was struggling with addiction. When I went to rehab and met other addicts, I was surrounded by people who were decades older than me. Although I could relate to them to a certain extent, the challenges you face as a young addict are often different than those as an older addict. While my peers were speaking of marriage, divorce, children, and career transitions, I was speaking about school, friends, and internships. I had not crossed the bridges that they had yet, nor did I feel anywhere close with my addiction getting in the way.

I began using at twenty and stopped by the age of twenty-two. You may be wondering what qualifies me to tackle such a hefty topic with only two years of using under my belt. After keeping my addiction secret for one year, coming clean to my family, attending addiction counselling, going to rehab, relapsing, and joining an anonymous fellowship of addicts, I have quite a lot to say. While addiction is certainly not glamorous, I am thankful for all that I have learned from the experience. Now that I am in recovery, I can look back and reflect on my time in active addiction and share my experiences with others who are struggling with similar issues. Addiction is far from one size fits all; however, there are many things that us addicts have in common.

Being a young addict, I am grateful that I have my whole life ahead of me to recover. Recovery is a lifelong process, and even though I am clean, my recovery process is far from over. Realizing your addiction and treating it early is a gift, because you still have your entire future ahead of you. The earlier you catch your addiction, the more time you have left to enjoy a life without substances.

I am especially grateful for my friends, family, and partner who have stuck by my side throughout the entire journey. It was not easy on any of us, yet we conquered it together. Not everyone has the support system that I did going through my addiction, and I hope this book helps those people feel less alone. Addiction is difficult on everyone involved, but it *is* possible to recover.

During active addiction, I lost a huge part of myself that I felt I could never get back, so I continued using. It wasn't until I stopped using that I realized substances were the problem and not the solution. People use substances for many reasons, but what ties us together are the underlying thoughts and feelings we experience as addicts. Lots of guilt and shame overtook my life when I was using substances, and now that I am clean, I can continue to piece myself together again, one step at a time.

Committing to sobriety for the rest of your life can seem daunting, so one of the first lessons I learned in rehab was to take things one day at a time. Rather than "for the rest of my life", we learned to focus just on today. This approach helped me tackle my fear of sober living. After using substances as a coping mechanism for almost two years, retraining my brain has not been easy, but necessary. When I just focus on today, recovery seems more tangible.

Even though we are addicts, we are not defined by our addiction. One mistake I made during my using days was just that. Addiction defined me and the way I lived my life. At first, I thought I was choosing substances, but soon the substances chose me. I lost control over myself and my life. I felt I had nowhere to go but downwards.

The reality is, we *can* go upwards. Addiction *can* be treated. Although there is no magic cure, hard work and dedication go a long way. Most addicts cannot do this on their own, which is why various treatment options exist. I highly encourage any addict who wants to get clean to take advantage of as many of these resources as possible, in order to assist you in your recovery. The bottom line is, you have to want recovery for yourself in order to succeed.

When I first began my recovery process, I was doing

it for other people rather than myself. I felt like a burden on my loved ones and felt that others were paying the price for my moral failing. However, addiction is not a moral failure, and it is nobody's fault. Just like cancer patients are not blamed for being diagnosed with cancer, addicts should not be blamed for their addiction. Many people are under the misconception that addiction is the product of bad life choices. However, many people make the same "bad" life choices and do not become addicts. This is because addiction is a disease, and it should be treated like any other illness.

If you are an addict, you are not alone. I hope this book serves as a useful resource for addicts and their loved ones to learn more about addiction. By exploring what addiction is, who addicts are, the consequences of addiction, what withdrawal is, what recovery is, how to deal with relapse, available treatment options, life without drugs, why to stop using now, friendships as a recovering addict, how to speak to loved ones about addiction, and how loved ones can help, I hope to provide additional clarity about addiction, who it affects, and how to best support loved ones suffering from addiction. This is by no means an exhaustive guide to addiction; however, I hope it benefits readers by providing a sense of solidarity to young addicts and their families.

My name is Katelyn, and I am an addict.

Chapter 1
What is Addiction, Anyways?

If you're like me in my early days of using, you may wonder if you are really an addict. After all, the term is not one size fits all. Addiction means many things to many people, and it can be confusing trying to determine exactly where you fall on the spectrum. You may consider yourself a recreational user, a stoner, or a partier, but in some way or other, substances are a part of your life. You may even consider yourself a "responsible user", yet it is important to remember there is no way to use substances safely.

When I began smoking marijuana, it started off occasional. A joint here, a joint there, mostly in social situations. I didn't realize that I had a problem until I began smoking weed on my own, at every hour of every day. Even then, I was just a "stoner", right? That was a lifestyle choice. Soon, however, weed was not something I was choosing any more; it was something that chose me. It was something I depended on to cope with the struggles of my everyday life. And soon, when weed wasn't enough, I began trying other chemical mechanisms that led me further and further away from myself, and further and further into the grasp of addiction.

It's easy to believe, at least at first, that substances are helping you. They may reduce your stress or give you energy when you're feeling down. They may give you strength or confidence or inner peace. It took me a long time and lots of therapy to realize that these illusions are just that — illusions. As a university student, "downers" like marijuana helped me unwind at the end of long, tireless days. At first, it truly did give the illusion of being helpful. My grades were never better than they had been in my early days of using, and I attributed that success to the ability of weed to help me slow down and step outside of myself, even if only temporarily, in order to reset my clock for the next strenuous day ahead. Soon, however, weed did start slowing me down, and "uppers" like cocaine offered a solution. Again, my grades skyrocketed, and I was convinced that these substances helped me be the best version of myself possible. Yet, over time, I lost a lot of money, time, friends, and most importantly, myself. I was no longer the one in control of my life.

Consuming substances — or rather, being consumed by substances — wasn't something I identified as problematic until a person very close to me expressed concern. I was high twenty-four hours a day, seven days a week; getting myself into dangerous situations, and even going to university under the influence. The stress when I would run out of my substance of choice was immense, and I would wait for what seemed like hours for my dealer to deliver my instant gratification. And the next day, it would all repeat.

As I mentioned before, addiction is not one size fits

all, and your story may differ from mine. However, there are a few common threads to consider when asking yourself if you have a substance use disorder.

First, do you use alone? Although taking substances at parties and with friends is something that is often normalized in youth culture, and even considered a regular "phase" that people our age experience, using alone is a sign that you are no longer in control. It wasn't until I realized that I didn't have to use with others that my dependence on substances truly began.

Second, have you used one drug as substitution for another, or used one drug to override the negative after-effects of the other? If the answer is yes, you may be creating a dependence on substances to cope with the harsh reality that your drug of choice is harming you, rather than helping you. When marijuana eventually began to take its negative toll on my grades, I patched up the issue with cocaine. When my obsession with cocaine began to turn me away from my studies, I resorted to more cocaine to "fix" the issue. Of course, it was never truly fixed and my so-called "success" at school was not because of my own doing; it was due to the help of mind-altering chemicals. In that way, I was no better than an athlete using steroids to achieve the next level of physical victory.

Finally, are drugs the first thing you go to in the morning and the last thing you go to before sleep? When I was in active addiction, substances were the first and last thoughts of my every day. I would use morning, noon, and night, craving the satisfaction substances provided me. And, when I ran out, a huge surge of anxiety would overcome me.

Of course, there are several other warning signs that you may be suffering from addiction. For example, putting substances ahead of financial responsibilities or relationships, trying to stop and not being able to, getting into dangerous situations because of substances, including legal trouble, blackouts, and overdosing, amongst others. If you follow a twelve-step program, the first step teaches you that you are powerless over your addiction or substance of choice. This means you no longer are in control, and substances have overcome your life. They take top priority over paying bills, studying, or hanging out with friends, on top of other important responsibilities. Drugs are isolating and all-consuming, and if you are reading this, they have likely become a bigger part of your life than you ever anticipated or wanted.

The first time I used cocaine was to celebrate a big accomplishment of mine, which, as mentioned before, I attributed to using marijuana. However, marijuana had become such a normal part of my life that I no longer felt the high I desired. So, I decided to try cocaine for the first time. I thought, "It's just one time, nothing will ever happen." — I couldn't have been more wrong. It quickly spiraled out of control, and within months, I was in a treatment center for addiction.

It's essential to realize that even though you may use drugs to regain control in your life that you feel you have lost, drugs will eventually betray you. Mind- and mood-altering substances offer a quick fix to deep, underlying issues we may not want to face, or may not know how to face. Just as quickly as drugs become the solution, however, they can become the problem. When using drugs, we are treating the symptoms, not the cause. In other words, we are self-medicating in order to numb certain feelings or emotions, but not the underlying causes of these feelings or emotions. It's easy to fall prey to the idea that substances can help us cope with traumatic events, mental disorders, stress, or even boredom — but by the time we realize that this may not be the case, we are already trapped in the cycle of addiction.

Addiction is defined in many ways, and the examples listed above are by no means exhaustive. The American Psychiatric Association (APA) defines addiction as a complex disease of the brain that is exhibited by the uncontrollable urge to use substances, despite negative repercussions. They proceed by emphasizing that people suffering from addiction (also known as a substance use disorder) have an intense compulsion to use substances to the point where it takes over their life.

It is important to note that addiction is not only characterized by drug abuse, but also alcohol abuse. It is common for people to think that because alcohol is legal, it is not "bad" or addictive. Unfortunately, that is not the case. Alcohol is, in fact, one of the most dangerous substances you can use and one of the most dangerous substances to stop using.

When I began my university studies, I was under the misconception that there was nothing wrong with drinking large amounts of alcohol. I would go to friends' houses to pre-drink, go to the pub for more drinks, then end up at a club and have even more drinks. While I should have taken this as a warning sign of addiction, I justified my drinking as a social and cultural activity that all of my peers took part in. What I didn't realize was that alcohol is a drug, just like every other substance. The misconception that it is not stems from its legality and commonplaceness in the everyday world. In other words, it is socially acceptable and easily accessible. However, we must be cognizant of its addictive abilities despite these misconceptions and do our best to stay away as addicts.

In fact, there are many common misconceptions about addiction. People think that addicts are "junkies" and that we all live under bridges sticking needles in our arms. While that is the case for some addicts, it is certainly not the case for all. It is possible to give off the impression that you are a functioning young adult while still being addicted to substances. In my case, no one pegged me as an addict, and when I told the people closest to me about my disorder, they were shocked. I dressed well, I was a university student, I had my own apartment. How could someone so seemingly "put together" be addicted?

The truth is, like people, addiction comes in many shapes and sizes. There is no way to "look like an addict". Just as someone living with a mental disability like turrets may not look "disabled", no one can tell if you are an addict just by looking at you. In fact, addicts often go through great lengths to hide their addiction from others. This may include hiding liquor bottles from partners or spraying copious amounts of perfume on their clothing to hide the smell of marijuana. Whatever it is, you cannot judge an addict just by looking at them. No matter how addicts are portrayed in the news and media, we aren't all the same.

Another misconception is that addiction is black and white. You're either an addict or you're not. However, when you're in the middle of active addiction, you may feel like you're in a grey area. For example, although I realized I was using far more than I should be and that I was experiencing harmful consequences because of my using, I always compared myself to other people. Because I wasn't using as much as Bobby or Susie, it must not be that bad, right? Or, because I wasn't using certain drugs, I didn't have a "real" problem, right? Wrong. Because addiction is not one-size fits all, you cannot compare yourself to other people.

You also can't compare the substances you use to the substances used by other people. Weed, for instance, is generally considered to be a relatively harmless and non-addictive drug. In university, I had many friends who frequently smoked weed. What I didn't realize was that, like any other drug, weed can be addictive. While it may not be considered "chemically" addictive like cocaine or heroin, it can be emotionally addictive, and for someone who was dealing with a lot of emotional issues at the time, I learned that the hard way. Just because you are using substance x and Bobby is using a "much worse" substance, substance y, this does not mean that you are not an addict.

Similarly, you cannot compare the length of time you have been using to someone else. It is easy to believe that you are not an addict because you have only been using for x amount of time. However, this is not cause to say that you are not an addict. Although I was fortunate enough to "only" have used for two years before getting clean, this does not mean I am not an addict. Everybody's path of addiction is different, and some people may be addicted for their entire lives, while other people are for only a portion. Simply stated, we cannot generalize one person's using experience to all users.

That said, addiction may be especially difficult to discern if you are a young woman, like myself. In the past, research into addiction focused only on males' use of drugs and alcohol. Until the 1990s, this exclusionary bias reflected how women were not seen as the addiction "type". Addiction was a male issue. However, since then, women have been included in more and more addiction studies. While research does indicate that you are almost two times more likely to be an addict if you are a male, females are more likely to be admitted to the hospital, and to fatally overdose.

Everything said, addiction can be difficult to gage if you are a young person. First, life itself seems complicated and confusing, and adding the possibility of addiction to the mix might make matters even more unclear. Especially because, as a young people, most of us are under the impression that only older adults can be addicts. Because we haven't been using for as long or are not as "experienced", we must not be addicts. This is faulty logic. Just because there may not be as many young people in rehab or in anonymous addiction fellowships does not mean they do not exist. It merely means that we are fortunate enough to have realized our addiction at an early stage, which is a good thing! Overcoming your addiction may be the hardest thing you've ever done or will ever have to do, but catching it is the first step to recovery.

Although scary, admitting you are an addict can also be empowering. For the first time in a long time, you have gained some control back. The substance is no longer using you the way it used to. Sure, you may not be able to stop using the first time you try, or the second time, or even the third time. These habits are quick to form and take a lifetime to change. But there is help out there. Addiction counselors, anonymous addiction fellowships, and inpatient as well as outpatient treatment centers are all possibilities.

Each step in the right direction will be challenging, but nothing worth doing is ever easy. Being frightened is natural. For the first time, you may be considering coping with life without the support of substances. For many people, substances offer the support that they feel they are lacking in their everyday lives. Unfortunately, many people may not know that you are lacking this support unless you come clean about your addiction.

When I told my family and friends what was going on with me, I was terrified — but also relieved. I finally didn't have to hide this part of myself and go through my addiction alone. Of course, not everyone in my situation may have the same support. That's exactly why anonymous addiction fellowships, counseling, and treatment centers exist. There are different options available depending on your personal needs and financial abilities. Just remember you are not the only one. Other addicts you meet — whether on the street, in school, or in treatment — are going through similar struggles to you. We are not all the same, but we have a lot in common. We are one-of-a-kind through our experiences as addicts.

Chapter 2
Who is an Addict, Anyways?

Just as addicts live to use, many of us must use to live. In other words, addiction has such a tight hold on us that we cannot physically or mentally survive without our substance of choice. When I read this, I assume that it must be a requirement to have used my entire life in order to "qualify" for addiction. While it is commonly misconceived that addicts are older adults, with several years of heavy using under their belts, addicts come in all ages. Many studies suggest that adolescents who begin using drugs or alcohol before the age of eighteen make up ninety percent of addicts in the United States. As part of the remaining ten percent, I can also say that using before the age of eighteen is not a requirement to become an addict. However, it does increase your chances. In fact, the most likely population to use drugs in the United States are Americans between the ages of eighteen and twenty-five. In the European Union, eighteen percent of sixteen-year-old students have used illicit substances at least once. This percentage varies significantly from country to country. For example, in the Czech Republic, this figure is more than double (thirty-seven percent). In my case, the stress of university, mental illness, and changes in the family all contributed to my first taste of drugs at the age of twenty. As you can see, addiction is not just an "adult" issue. It affects adolescents and young adults just as much.

Equally important, addiction affects all genders. As a young adult woman, in particular, I felt left out of addiction. I believed that I was a rare case, because everyone else that I knew who used were men. While it is more common for men to use than women, female addicts are out there, we just may be harder to find due to research biases that are still being overcome, in addition to the shame of feeling like we are one of the only female addicts around. It wasn't until I went to rehab that I realized as a woman, I am not alone. Addiction affects all genders, as does any other disease like coronavirus, cancer, or the common cold.

Interestingly, however, studies suggest that some people may be more predisposed to becoming addicted than others. This is because of genetics. It is believed that if you come from a family with a history of addiction, you are more likely to become an addict yourself than if you do not come from a family with a history of addiction. In fact, the APA estimates that approximately fifty percent of addiction comes down to genetics. While this is still being researched to establish more concrete evidence, I am the loved one of an addict, and two of my relatives have died from overdose. The facts may only be correlational at this point, but it is important to be aware of your family history when picking up drugs for the first time. Ideally, no one would. However, people do for various reasons, and some manage to get addicted, while others don't. This theory offers one possible explanation as to why.

Another theory is that addiction is a combination of nature and nurture. In other words, addiction is both the result of genetics, or who we are on the inside, and the environment we find ourselves in on the outside. Although not everyone who is predisposed to addiction and going through stressful life events will become an addict, when we combine the two, addiction is even more likely.

What's most imperative to realize is that while we all have our own reasons for getting involved with drugs, no one chooses to get addicted. In fact, most of us think, "that'll never be me". No one picks up their first joint or takes their first drink thinking, "I'm going to be an addict." It's human nature to minimize possibilities like this. Otherwise, how would we cope with the fear of everyday life? Most people don't leave their house thinking, "I'm going to get into a car accident today." But unfortunately, some do. Rather than assume the worst, humans tend to assume the best.

Although you cannot predict addiction, many addicts have some personality traits in common. These include, but are not limited to: impulsivity, "all or nothing" thinking, compulsivity, obsession, grandiosity, perfectionism, low self-esteem, nonconformity, stress, mental illness and denial. You do not have to tick every box to be an addict, or you may tick even more. As stated before, everyone is different, but we are tied together by some common threads.

Impulsivity refers to impulsive behavior, or behavior which you feel you cannot control. For example, you may act on an impulse rather than thinking something through. For me, impulsivity comes in the form of constantly wanting instant gratification. When I submit an essay in school, I want the grade back right away. When I see something that I like at the store, I must buy it now. If I had a craving for a drug, I gave in every time, despite negative repercussions as a result. Even today, I lack long-term perspective and always focus on the short-term consequences of my actions. This is impulsivity.

Similarly, "all or nothing" thinking refers to one's inability to find balance in their behaviors, whether it be exercising, spending money, dieting, or using substances. Somebody with an all or nothing attitude will either go one-hundred and ten percent at the gym every day or never go at all. There is no healthy balance in "all or nothing" thinkers' lives, no such thing as moderation. In my case, I am either all in or all out. It's black or it's white. There is no such thing as treating myself to a piece (or two) of chocolate after a long day of schoolwork. I either eat healthy for the entire day, or I binge eat as much as I can before the day is over, so I can start over again the next day. "All or nothing" thinkers are very prone to addiction because we cannot control our impulses except to the extremes. This is very unhealthy, no matter which area of life this behavior applies to.

Compulsivity is the need or desire to perform behaviors repeatedly in a difficult-to-break cycle. It is easy to conceive how drugs fall into this picture. I, for example, exhibit mild symptoms of obsessive-compulsive disorder. If I do something as simple as turn a doorknob, I must do it an even number of times before

I feel completely satisfied. Some drugs actually feed into compulsivity, such as cocaine. It tricks your brain into wanting more, and more, and more, until you have no more lines to take. Its chemical composition induces cravings and makes it difficult to stop after just one. So, you have one after the other, after the other, and you still have the urge to take even more. Taking drugs in this way greatly increases your chance of overdose and shows just how easy it is to fall into a cycle of substance abuse.

Obsession is the tendency to obsess over thoughts, feelings, or events that you experience in your life. In other words, it is a major preoccupation with someone or something. Obsession is common in addicts, who obviously obsess over substance use, but also other activities too, such as eating, exercising, relationships, or schoolwork. In addition to previously obsessing over substances, I tend to obsess over school, work, and most of all, myself. In fact, self-obsession is very common in addicts. Similar to grandiosity, this means we are constantly preoccupied with ourselves and often unconcerned about others. For example, our self-obsession may take the shape of bragging or apathy. The world revolves around us, and we revolve around substances.

Grandiosity is a sense of egocentricity or superiority exhibited by an individual. Someone who is grandiose and engaging in substance use for the first time may think that they have a stronger willpower than the average person, and therefore will never become an addict. While willpower is certainly a valuable skill to have, it is useless in treating addiction. I stopped using drugs temporarily several times before I finally realized I needed more than just willpower to quit. Without proper treatment, it is nearly impossible to stop using with one's willpower alone. Quitting using mind and mood-altering substances requires a complete lifestyle change, similar to dieting. If you only have willpower, you will be able to resist several temptations that will eventually build up, and in the end, you will give in to that slice of cake.

Perfectionism refers to one's inability to accept any standard other than 'perfect.' Perfectionists are often very hard on themselves and engage in much self-criticism. As a perfectionist, I put huge pressure on myself to achieve highly. In order to manage this stress, I used to use substances. When my results would come back even a millimeter shy of perfect, I would put even more pressure on myself to perform 'perfectly' the next time. As a result of this enormous stress, I would use again. Each time, I would try to prove to myself that I was good enough, setting unrealistically high standards, inevitably failing, and getting caught in a cycle of never being happy with myself or my accomplishments. From there, the cycle of perfectionism continued, with addiction alongside it. What everyone must remember is that perfection does not exist. Nobody can be perfect, no matter how hard you try. It is unrealistic to put such high standards on yourself, and it is even more unrealistic to translate these standards onto others, which addicts also often do. Using as a result of perfectionism reflects very low-levels of self-esteem and keeps the cycle going until you begin to accept that your aims are beyond reach. Sometimes, good enough is good enough.

Low self-esteem is characterized by a poor self-image. People with low self-esteem may be able to project an air of confidence, yet lack it in reality. For a long time, I masked my low self-esteem with substances. My sense of perfectionism originates from a well-ingrained fear that I will never be good enough. I will never be smart enough to get a job, or worthy enough to be loved. I will never be thin enough to be beautiful. The list goes on. When I discovered drugs, I also discovered a new sense of self that was numb to all of these toxic beliefs, a sense of self that I thought was made better by drugs. However, the tables eventually turned, and the reason for my low self-esteem became my addiction. I went from thinking I was not smart, worthy, or beautiful to also thinking I was not worth getting clean for. Although substances are often characterized by their positive effects on the mind, the negative, long-term effects are often overlooked.

Nonconformity is the refusal to follow certain rules or customs. This manifests in addicts, who oftentimes believe they do not need to follow societal practices. Growing up as somewhat of an outcast, I developed a sense of nonconformity early on. I didn't understand why things had to be done a certain way, and I believed my way was best. I quickly outgrew societal norms and practices with the desire to be different or "edgy". Tattoos, cigarettes, alcohol, and eventually other drugs took over my life. I didn't have to conform to society if I didn't want to. To an extent, my nonconformity stems from my sense of grandiosity, thinking I am above the law or that I am "special" or "different." Truth be told, I am no different than any other addict, and I am no better than any other person. Nonconformity was a facade I was wearing in order to mask some of my deeper issues.

Stress also plays a large role in addiction. Many — if not most — addicts have in common a huge burden of stress on their shoulders. Of course, not all people who are stressed become addicts. Certain amounts of stress are necessary in order for humans to function. However, too much stress and the inability to cope with it all, whether it be financial, familial, or in any other form, can lead to unhealthy habits. I first started using heavily in university. For the first two years I managed to handle my stress in healthy ways, such as going to the gym. However, by my third year many stressful events had compounded, and the only way I saw out was substances. Learning to deal with stress in productive ways takes time. It is not easy to change well-ingrained coping mechanisms overnight. However, it is essential for recovery. Stress will always be there; what can change it is the way we choose to tackle it.

Mental illness also plays a significant role in addiction. Mental illness is a condition that affects one's health and is characterized by thinking, emotional, and/or behavioral shifts. Examples include depression, anxiety, bipolar disorder, and schizophrenia. According to the American Psychiatric Association, approximately twenty percent of adults in the United States experience some type of mental illness in their lifetime. Of these adults, one in twelve meet the criteria for a comorbid substance use disorder. However, several studies have suggested that substance use can lead to the onset of certain mental illnesses, like schizophrenia. So, it is unclear whether mental illness brings on using, or if using brings on mental illness. Both are likely to be true. From my own experience living with bipolar disorder, it was easier to turn to substances to balance out my sporadic moods and behavior than to learn to cope with the inconsistency myself. When I was manic, I would use downers to relax me, and when I was depressive, I would use uppers to bring me back up. For a long time, this worked, and I felt like I was living a stable life — until the financial difficulties, the school difficulties, and the relationship difficulties began to accompany my using. Although self-medicating provided a temporary solution to my condition, in the long-term it made things much worse. When coming down from drugs, I would feel even worse than I had before I had taken them. I felt huge amounts of guilt and shame at what I had just done. When the substances wore off, I was in the same place in my life that I was before I took them; my problems didn't just disappear. Although much stigma still exists around mental illness and addiction, it is common for the two to go hand in hand. Luckily, different therapies and medications are available to help treat mental illness and addiction in productive ways.

Finally, denial refers to the rejection of something that is true. I saved this characteristic for last because I figured some of you may be reading this book thinking, "No, this isn't me. I don't have a problem." That is exactly what an addict in denial would say. They might continue denying they have a problem, continue using, and continue excusing their behavior because they are convinced that they are fine. When I was in the deepest depths of my addiction, I almost lost my relationship because of this mentality. Denying an issue does not mean it does not exist. The issue is still there, but the will to change it is not. Recovery begins with jumping over the hurdle of denial into a state of acceptance. *Yes, I am addicted. And yes, I need help.*

Again, these characteristics are not universal to all addicts everywhere. However, they are common traits that we possess. Some people, like myself, might tick all of these boxes. Some may tick only a few. Some may tick even more that are not mentioned here. What is important to grasp is that us addicts are not alone in our thoughts and feelings. Although we all come from different backgrounds, many of the feelings underlying our unique experiences are the same.

It was not until I went to rehab that I realized these similarities. While many of the people in my treatment center had experienced events that I had not, such as spending time in prison as a result of their addiction, our group therapy sessions unveiled that we all shared an overwhelming sense of guilt and shame about our addictions. No one asks to be an addict, and no one wants to be an addict. The guilt and shame were the result of the failure we felt to live a "normal" life, the effects we had on our loved ones, and overall disappointment in ourselves. Growing up, I was always the "perfect" child. I didn't argue with my parents, I got good grades, and I was always very involved in extracurricular activities. Addiction was never something I imagined in my future. Guilt and shame are normal to experience as an addict, and if you feel those too, you are certainly not alone.

Addiction may not be the same for everyone — we may be addicted to different substances, have different reasons for using, use it for different periods of time, or be different ages, genders, races or religions — but that is exactly the point. Addiction spans across all backgrounds and cultures. Many people still view addiction as a personal fault; however, more and more people are beginning to accept that addiction is a disease, not just the result of "bad" or "stupid" decisions. The fifth edition of the Diagnostic and Statistical Manual (DSM-5), established by the American Psychiatric Association to define and classify mental disorders, now includes substance use disorders in their volume. This is huge progress, as substance use is now being treated like any other disorder and not merely the fault of the addict. With time, we can hope that stigma will continue to decrease, and knowledge about addiction will continue to increase. More extensive research will be done and more effective treatments developed.

Even throughout human history, beliefs about substances have fluctuated. For example, multiple substances have been historically used by different cultures for healing and celebratory purposes. Cocaine used to be an active ingredient in Coca-Cola, which was advertised as an intellectual brain-booster. Opioids and alcohol used to be used to treat pain during the Revolutionary War. Hemp, whose fibers were used for fabric, paper, and rope, stemmed from marijuana, and eventually the substance extended into recreational use. Over time, however, the dangers of these substances were realized, and the use of drugs and alcohol went from celebrated to scolded. Reports of psychosis and the misconception that substance use led to violence and criminality prompted this response.

To this day, attitudes are constantly changing regarding substance use. Marijuana, for example, is being legalized again in many places. It is decriminalized in many others. While this may be disconcerting if you are a fellow marijuana addict, it goes to show how approaches to substances and substance use change over time. This does not mean you should go to your local dispensary and buy a joint to celebrate how far humanity has come. Always be wary that weed can be addictive too. However, as addicts, we should celebrate the changing mindset towards the treatment of addiction and the de-stigmatization of our disease.

The moral of the story is this: despite the stereotypes of addicts being lazy, unmotivated, or violent lowlifes, we are people, just like everybody else. Everybody faces their own challenges in life. While others may not fully understand addiction yet, what is most important is that you understand your own addiction and take the steps needed towards your recovery. Do not worry what others think of you. What matters is what you think of yourself. This will improve as you venture further and further into recovery, and further and further away from chemical dependence.

Chapter 3
What are the Consequences of Addiction, Anyways?

When asked about drugs, many people will make an association with crime. Cocaine, heroin, weed, and any other illegal substances are synonymous with time behind bars. Alcohol, on the other hand, is associated with fun, socializing, or relaxing after a long day at work. Why the difference? Mere legality? Although alcohol may escape this substance-stereotype, the consequences of alcoholism are no different than any other drug addiction.

While prison time is a possible consequence of being caught using, possessing, or selling substances, drugs have unfairly been associated with criminality since the decline of legal, recreational use. Although most drugs are illegal in most places around the world, users do not become inherently "criminal" or "dangerous" just by using them. While it is true that certain drugs may incline some people to act more violently, riskily, or engage in criminal activity, most people do not experience this. For example, someone may think they are capable of driving a car under the influence of alcohol, or someone may become irrationally angry or abusive under the influence of stimulants. In these cases, authorities may get involved not only to protect the individual under the influence, but also the people around them. What to take from this is that while some people may exhibit dangerous behavior under the influence, drugs themselves do not cause violence.

When I was regularly using substances, I was lucky enough to never face any legal action. However, many people do face time in prison as a result of their addiction. Whether this is from mere possession, the intention to sell/distribute, or dangerous behavior, prison can have profound and long-lasting effects on incarcerated individuals. As someone who has worked in prisons in the United States, I know this from experience speaking with incarcerated people. Prison can be detrimental not only to mental health while incarcerated, but also following incarceration. Especially in places like the United States, where having a criminal record repeals your right to vote, many employment opportunities, many educational opportunities, and the ability to find housing. However, these issues are not exclusive to the United States. Many of these "side-effects" translate across borders, and can make life very difficult for released, recovering individuals. As previously established, stress and the environment you find yourself in are huge factors that influence addiction.

For example, if Joe is released from jail after five years and cannot find a job, decent housing, or get an education, what kind of future does he have in front of him? A pretty bleak one. This may only encourage the use of substances even more. While some countries, like Sweden, do take a more rehabilitative approach to crime (including drug offenses) rather than a punitive one, the exact consequences you face depend on where in the world you are living. Besides, not all substances are treated equally under the law. In Sweden, individuals convicted of a minor drug offense (i.e., possession of a small amount) are exposed to fines or up to six months imprisonment in a dorm-like facility. Swedish officials report that their prisons have small populations, and that incarcerated individuals are encouraged to re-enter society in better shape than when they entered the facility. In comparison, individuals convicted of a minor drug offense in the United States (called simple possession), can face fines and much longer in prison in an overcrowded facility where retribution is the goal. This goes to show two very different approaches to correcting drug offenses. Ideally, no one would get involved with drugs in the first place. However, without proper support inside or outside of prisons (no matter where in the world you are), breaking the cycle of addiction can be very difficult.

Another possible consequence of addiction is adverse health effects. Using substances can cause damage to the respiratory system, cardiovascular system, digestive system, liver, kidney, and brain. It can also lead to infectious diseases such as HIV and Hepatitis, increased risk of overdose and withdrawal, and have negative prenatal effects on unborn babies.

Let's start with the respiratory system. Substances that you snort, such as cocaine, MDMA, and meth, can cause irreversible damage to the nose. This includes damage to soft tissues and holes in the nasal cavity. While snorting drugs is not always the fastest way to feel drugs' effects, it can prolong the high felt from certain drugs, such as cocaine. Minor nasal consequences of snorting substances may be a runny or bloody nose, indicative of a sinus infection. However, if you engage in snorting more often, the infected tissues may not have proper time to heal between uses, and more serious problems can develop. Likewise, substances that you smoke cause damage to the lungs after prolonged periods of time. Many people choose to smoke their drug of choice due the rapid onset of desired effects. Lung cancer, bronchitis, emphysema, chronic obstructive pulmonary disease (COPD), lung damage, respiratory problems, slowed breathing, and worsening asthma are all negative effects that can result from inhaled substances (even tobacco!). During my heaviest period of using, I was smoking around five to six joints per day. I noticed my general respiratory fitness decrease, and I developed a frequent cough. Yet, it is impossible to see the interior effect this had on my lungs. I may not know the consequence for years. If you haven't started smoking yet, it is a good idea never to. If you are currently smoking any kind of substance — even tobacco — it is advisable that you seek help and stop as soon as possible in order to prevent further damage. Although the lungs can repair themselves over time, the sooner you stop, the better your chances are.

Next, studies have shown that most drugs can have adverse effects on the cardiovascular system. This includes the heart, veins, blood vessels and valves. These effects can range in severity, from an abnormal heart rate to a heart attack or stroke. Even smoking tobacco significantly increases one's chance of developing heart disease. Injection drug use can pose an even more concerning threat to the cardiovascular system, including the risk of collapsing veins and bacterial infections which affect the blood vessels and valves. HIV and hepatitis as a result of injecting substances can also lead to a heightened risk of liver-related morbidity and mortality. When I was using stimulants, I remember using so much that my heart felt like it was going to explode out of my chest. It would pulsate rapidly and with much more force than usual. Sometimes I would feel like I was having a panic attack, and I would have to lay down to control my breathing for what felt like forever until the high wore off. While it's easy for me to look back and recognize that this wasn't healthy for my body, in the midst of active addiction, it is easy to lack that perspective. Getting high takes top priority, and that comes with the negative side effects, too.

The digestive system is also affected when taking substances. Many can induce nausea and vomiting, even if only taken once. Specifically, cocaine is known to cause bowel decay and gum decay in the mouth. When I began using cocaine, I loved the feeling of numbness in my teeth. I didn't know that this was an effect of cocaine, and I also didn't know that it can cause severe deterioration of your gums. Once the gums have receded, they cannot grow back. Periodontitis (gum disease) is a great risk that cocaine users face. That said, any drug taken through the digestive tract can be harmful.

In addition, chronic use of certain drugs, such as

alcohol, heroin, inhalants, and steroids, can significantly impair the functioning of liver. In severe cases, the liver may even shut down entirely. Similarly, drugs can impair the functioning of the kidney and even lead to kidney failure. Drugs such as heroin, MDMA, steroids, bath salts and even tobacco do this through dangerous increases in body temperature, dehydration, and muscle breakdown. Severe damage to the liver or kidney can lead to death.

Finally, it's obvious that substances also affect the brain. We know this because of the euphoric effects we experience when we use. However, what most drug dealers won't tell you is that these substances can also cause extreme brain damage from seizures, stroke, and by damaging brain cells. If you've ever seen the 1987 anti-narcotics campaign by Partnership for a Drug Free America, you'll remember the image of an egg frying in a frying pan. Well, folks, although it may seem like an exaggeration, to an extent, this representation is accurate. When addiction occurs, repeated substance use causes changes to the brain's neurological pathways. This change in the brain's wiring alters how the brain controls stress, pleasure, impulse control, decision-making, and memory, amongst other important functions. This makes it even harder to tackle addiction, because you must re-train the way your brain works.

Because of all the stress your body is put under while using, every time you use a substance you are putting yourself at risk of overdose. As you begin using more regularly, you will begin to build up a tolerance for your substance of choice. Tolerance means it takes more and more of a substance to obtain its desired effects.

However, tolerance is a slippery slope to overdose if you're not careful about just how much you are putting into your body. Overdose is when you take too much of a drug that your body can't cope with. Signs of overdose include severe chest pain, severe headaches, seizures, difficulty breathing, delirium, anxiety, irregular pulse, extreme agitation, extreme changes in body temperature, and loss of consciousness. While it's not always easy to discern if somebody (including yourself) is overdosing or just experiencing the regular effects of a drug, if you suspect you or someone else is overdosing, call your local emergency number for help. Drug-related emergencies are not typically prosecuted by the police. The main goal of emergency services is to help the person in distress. By calling for help, you could be saving someone's life.

While overdose means that you have too much of a substance in your body, withdrawal means that you have too little of a substance in your body. Withdrawal happens when we become physiologically dependent on a drug and need it order for our bodies to function (see Chapter Four). When the drug is no longer present — for example, when we are trying to quit — our bodies often react by producing undesirable physical effects. These can range in severity from headaches to seizures. Although unpleasant, withdrawal symptoms are often unavoidable when trying to get clean.

Clearly, the health effects resulting from addiction are nothing short of scary. However, addicts are not the only ones who can be affected by substance use. Unborn babies of mothers who use substances during pregnancy are also at risk of developing problems. These negative prenatal effects include premature birth, miscarriage, behavioral or cognitive issues in the child growing up, and/or neonatal abstinence syndrome (when a baby is born dependent on a substance used by its mother during pregnancy). However, even if you know your baby is at risk, it is not easy to stop using substances. Addiction is a compulsive disease that encourages users to continue using, despite awareness of its negative repercussions.

For example, if you're like me, the risk of adverse health effects was not enough to get me to stop using. For me, the breaking point came when I almost lost my relationship, fell behind in school, and went broke. These effects may not cost you your life, but they put things into perspective because they are effects that you can actually see in front of you, as opposed to the effects going on inside of your body.

Relationships are tricky when you're suffering from an addiction. Your partner, family, and friends may not understand exactly what is going on with you. You may attend family events intoxicated, stop going out with your friends in order to use, or put drugs before spending time with your significant other. Whatever shape your addiction takes, it is not easy for non-addicts to understand addiction. My partner always complained that he felt like I loved drugs more than him. While that was not the case, drugs had such a hold on me that I felt I could not give them up, even for him. That's what's important to realize though: you have to want to quit drugs on your own, not just for someone else. Doing it for someone else isn't going to help you in the long run. It may offer short-term motivation, but when the times get tough, you will always fall back into the revolving door of addiction. You have to want sobriety for yourself in order to achieve your goals.

In addition to my relationship being put in jeopardy by drugs, I quickly fell behind in school once the "honeymoon period" of using was behind me. At first, substances helped me achieve my academic goals to a golden standard; however, with time they derailed my motivation, energy, and desire to succeed. I began skipping classes to use, going to the classes I did attend under the influence, missing deadlines, and eventually ended up withdrawing from my classes in order to avoid failing. Through all of this, I thought drugs were the only solution to pick me back up and put the pieces together again. It wasn't until I went to rehab that I realized my so-called "solution" had turned into the problem. If your academic work is suffering as a result of your addiction, your school should have resources that can help you, such as counseling. Many schools want to help their students with addiction, you just have to ask.

Finally, financial distress meant I was not able to sustain my using habits. When I first started off, I was not using as much and could afford the occasional "treat". However, as my addiction grew stronger, my self-control grew weaker, and I was spending upwards of two hundred and fifty euros per week on my addiction. Living off of student loans and unpaid internships, that was almost all of my weekly budget. My diet became pasta and eggs, and my social life deteriorated because I could no longer afford to go out with friends. I had to stop seeing the doctor when I was sick because I could no longer afford to. I had to start walking places, because I did not have the money to buy bus tickets. I had to call my dad and beg for money because "something came up" and I didn't have enough. Putting substances before your financial needs is indicative of addiction. Whether that means spending all of your money on drugs, losing your job, putting substances before paying your bills, being evicted from your house, or having your car repossessed, it all stems from the same underlying issue.

As you can see, the consequences of addiction are far from appealing. Prison time, adverse health effects, relationship problems, trouble at work or school, and financial difficulties are all part of the equation. If you haven't experienced all of these consequences yet, that doesn't mean you will not throughout the course of your addiction. Of course, if you're reading this book, I want nothing but success for you in your recovery. The purpose of this chapter was to inform both users and non-users of what can happen when addiction takes over. Recovery is not easy. However, when you begin to recover, you can also begin to put these broken pieces together again.

Chapter 4
What is Withdrawal, Anyways?

If you've ever used substances, chances are you may be familiar with the feeling of a comedown. Comedowns, or "crashes", refer to the decline in mood or energy you feel after using stimulants. Comedowns are anything but fun and can even last multiple days, depending on how heavily you use. For example, when I was using cocaine, I would feel extremely tired, irritable, anxious, and depressed for around one to three days after my binge took place. I didn't want to hang out with friends, I didn't want to go to school, and I didn't want to leave my bed (similar to a hangover). Comedowns are the result of a drug being cleared from your blood; although, traces of the drug can still be present in the blood for much longer.

Withdrawal is similar to a comedown, except much more severe. Withdrawal refers to the symptoms that result from abruptly arresting or reducing the consumption of your substance of choice. Because substances — whether it be alcohol, heroin, meth, or any other drug — have psychoactive effects on the brain, it is easy to develop physiological dependence. This means that users may require their substance of choice in order to function and feel "normal" in their everyday lives. When a user tries to stop or limit their intake, this dependence may translate into withdraw symptoms. These withdrawal symptoms are often very unpleasant and uncomfortable for the affected person.

By going through withdrawal, the body is trying to find its new balance, or homeostasis, without the drug present. For example, quitting "cold turkey", or immediately, means that there is substantially less of a drug in an addict's body. The sudden absence of its usual bodily concentration and chemical fluctuations in the brain manifests through several mental, emotional, and/or physical symptoms.

Common withdrawal symptoms include severe headaches, trembling, nausea, vomiting, insomnia (difficulty sleeping), anxiousness, easy agitation, excessive sweating, body aches, depression, hallucinations, lethargy, fluctuations in body temperature, and even seizures. Because of the severity of these symptoms, it can be dangerous to stop all at once. If you are at risk of withdrawal, it is best to talk to your doctor before trying to quit using on your own. Rather than quitting cold turkey, your doctor may want you to gradually ween off of substances or even go through a medical detox in order to manage your symptoms (see below).

In particular, alcohol is a very dangerous drug to stop using in one go. As I mentioned in Chapter One, alcohol is one of the most dangerous substances to use and one of the most dangerous substances to stop using. Its legality does not detract from this fact. Alcohol is a central nervous sytstem (CNS) depressent, meaning it slows you down. Abruptly stopping drinking alcohol can overly-excite the nervous system as the body restores its equilibrium. Mild symptoms may include headache, shaky hands, sweating, nasua, vomiting, anxiety, and insomnia. More serious symptoms may include confusion, racing heartbeat, high blood pressure, fever, hallucinations, delusions, and seizures. Some of these effects can present themselves within hours of one's last drink and last up to several days. It may even take weeks or longer to come off alcohol, or other addictive substances.

The severity and duration of an addict's withdrawal is dependent on several factors, such as which drug(s) they used, the amount they used, and the frequency of use. Generally speaking, the stronger the dependence an individual has on a drug, the worse their withdrawal symptoms will be. Symptoms can last from days to months and even years if not properly treated. That's why medical detox is recommended in many cases where an addict would like to come clean of substances.

Medical detox involves withdrawal management in a hospital or medical setting in order to ease the onset of symptoms and treat them where necessary. For many substances, this is the safest way to go about getting sober. For many people, this is the most comfortable way to go about getting sober. While in detox, medical professionals will monitor vital signs (such as body temperature and blood pressure) and treat severe symptoms with medication where needed. The ultimate goal of detox is to rid the body of substances while maintaining the highest possible level of safety and comfort in the patient. Addicts who use alcohol, opiods, benzodiazepines, and other sedative substances often benefit from medical detox.

When I was in rehab, all patients were put on detox for various amounts of time depending on which drugs they used, how much they used and when their last use was. Every night, the nurses would come in while we were sleeping to check our vitals and make sure everything was running smoothly, which would inevitably wake us up. Although annoying at the time, I am thankful for the dedicated team who made sure we were all stable, in case that anything went wrong. While I was only on detox for a week, many others were for several weeks, with more frequent checks of their vitals throughout the day. As I've reinforced throughout this book, addiction is not one size fits all. What is best for one person may not be best for another. So, approaches to treating withdrawal may vary.

At this point, you are probably wondering which substances have the worst withdrawals. You may think that depending on the substance you use, you will not have to worry about withdrawal. Unfortunately, this is not the case. Even marijuana, which has a reputation for being non-addictive and withdraw-free, is neither of those things. Despite misconceptions, marijuana withdrawal does exist. It may not be as severe as that of opioids, for example, but heavy, frequent users will likely experience some degree of withdrawal upon ceasing to use the drug. Withdrawal symptoms from marijuana include lack of appetite, mood swings, irritability, difficulty sleeping, changes in focus, cravings for the drug, sweating, chills, depression, and/or gastrointestinal problems.

Although I didn't realize it at the time, I likely suffered from marijuana withdrawal when I first stopped using. I lost a lot of weight, had intense cravings, difficulty falling asleep, and many gastrointestinal problems that, at the time, I did not attribute to marijuana withdrawal. With the legalization and decriminaliztion of marijuana taking place in many areas around the world, it is important that we debunk the existing myths about marijuana. Yes, it is addictive, and yes, it can cause withdrawal.

While an especailly harsh comedown or hangover may give you a brief taste of what it is like to withdrawal, withdrawal is much, much worse. Physical and mental symptoms often make it difficult — if not impossible — for individuals to function during the withdrawal period. Many individuals require medical detox and cannot do this on their own. If you are considering quitting your substance of choice, make sure you consult your doctor to make sure you do it in the safest and most comfortable way possible. It is better to be safe than sorry.

Although withdrawal is anything but fun, it may be necessary in order to begin your recovery. Don't let the discomfort of withdrawal symptoms dissuade you from getting clean. Remember, after all of the pain and malaise you may experience coming off of your substance of choice, you will be one step closer to the life you want to live. As I mention in the next chapter, recovery is a lifelong process, and it is far from easy. However, once you get past the initital stage of withdrawal, you will be in a better position to start living your life again, one sober step at a time.

Chapter 5
What is Recovery, Anyways?

If I had to sum up my experience in recovery in just a few words, it would be tumultuous, emotional, and the hardest thing I've ever done. Recovery, like anything in life, has its ups and downs. Some days are easier than others. Some days I'll be particularly stressed out about whatever cards I was dealt that day; some nights I'll have dreams about the life I've left behind now. Regardless of what tempts you to run towards substances, leaving them behind is difficult, but necessary.

Although there is no one definition of recovery, abstinence from substances is a requirement, including alcohol. Every recovering addict sees recovery through their own lens, and in this book, I hope to share mine with you. To me, recovery is not only the absence of substances, but the presence of support from other recovering addicts. I did not realize the importance of the latter until I went to rehab. I thought recovery was merely staying away from substances, but forming relationships with other recovering addicts is truly what saved me. It takes a village.

The beauty of forming bonds with other recovering addicts is that we understand each other. We don't have to explain why we use, or what we use, or how much we use, like we do to our family and friends who are trying to understand our addictions. We simply introduce ourself, say we are an addict, and a mutual understanding is born. We may not know every detail about these people's lives or using (at least at first), but that's not the point. The point is, we've all had experiences that have driven us to using, and now we all have experiences that are driving us to stop. Just like every addiction is not the same, neither is every recovery. However, many underlying thoughts, emotions, and fears are common between recovering addicts.

When I first walked through the doors of rehab some time ago, I was very skeptical about treatment. I built up a wall so no one could get through to the real me, including my counsellors and other patients. I didn't think rehab would work, and I didn't see why I had to be stuck in a building with other addicts in order to recover. Wasn't that counterintuitive? Wouldn't the shared experience of using make me want to use even more? Surprisingly, no. The community I felt in rehab, no matter how closed off I was at the beginning, was very welcoming and genuine.

At first, I thought it was fake. I thought the other patients had been brainwashed by the nurses and that I was entering a house of horrors to meet my demise. All of the other patients spoke so highly of the place when I first arrived — I thought they must be mad to be so happy to be there. As a university student, rehab was definitely not my first choice of places to spend my spring break. However, with time, I realized I hadn't given treatment a fair chance. If I was closed off to treatment, of course it wouldn't work, because I wouldn't let it. I went from a patient labelled as "difficult" to a patient with their eyes wide open, and finally, I began to benefit from the greatness the other patients spoke about.

Don't get me wrong, rehab was not fun, and I have absolutely no desire to go back. However, I learned a lot about myself and my addiction from the experience. Had I not gone, I may not be in the same place I am today. Through all the meltdowns, tearful phone calls home, and emotional therapy sessions, I came out alive and stronger. And, most importantly, not alone. The strongest, most candid friendships I've ever made came out of that once-frightening facility, and I couldn't be more grateful for the amazing personalities I met during my time there. Without the support of other people who were in my position and time clean under my belt, my recovery experience would have been very different.

Of course, rehab is not the only option available to recovering addicts. For many reasons, rehab may not be a possibility for everyone. Even if you do go to rehab, you will still need support once you leave. That's why there's also addiction counseling and anonymous addiction fellowships for people who are either in recovery or wish to be in recovery. While I would certainly recommend addiction counseling from my own experience, the benefit of joining an anonymous addiction fellowship is that you get to meet other recovering addicts. Having a sense community is what has really helped me overcome my addiction. By nature, I am a very shy and introverted person; yet, the people I have met in treatment have made me comfortable enough to come out of my shell. Anonymous addiction fellowships can be an outlet when you feel you have nowhere else to go. No one is there to judge; they just listen and relate.

Recovery may seem scary at first, because it is a lifelong commitment to sobriety. Oftentimes, we are not able to succeed on our first go, especially if we are not receiving proper treatment. We may quit on willpower alone, and when it breaks, we go back to our substance of choice. We may quit for good, but use "just one last time" as a farewell ode to our "friend", quickly turned foe. We may use at a party or social event, making the mistake of thinking we can be "recreational" users. No matter how it goes down, relapse isn't fun. It may be until the effect of the drugs wear off, but once they do, you've hit rock bottom. Again. And this time, it's worse. If you've spent time trying to get clean and change your habits, relapsing can be extremely frustrating, embarrassing, and defeating. The overwhelming sense of guilt and shame you felt before trying to quit comes back ten times stronger, because you thought you were making progress.

Even though you may want to blame yourself, remember that giving up substances forever is not achieved overnight. When our bodies are going through so much change, it is natural for the cravings to come along. It is natural for our brains to want to revert back to the only coping mechanism they know — chemicals. It takes time for this automatic response to be overridden. However, as time goes on, these cravings will get less and less frequent and easier and easier to deal with.

When I began writing this book, I thought relapse was important to write about because it was a natural part of many addicts' recoveries. However, I learned from a wise man that actually, relapse isn't part of recovery; it is a part of addiction. It is our disease trying to resurface through all of our efforts to stay clean. That said, if you relapse, that does not mean you are failing. In fact, relapse means you are trying, really, really hard. Relapsing is the body's way of trying to comfort itself through such a shock to its system — the realization that it's not running on substances any more. If you've relapsed, don't give up on your recovery or think less of yourself. This is just another hurdle to overcome. Accept what happened, forgive yourself, and move on with your recovery. It may be tempting to use again in order to numb the shame of relapsing the first time — but don't fall for this illusion. Drugs are deceptive, and unfortunately thinking they will solve the problem is part of our disease.

What helps me in my recovery is remembering to take things one day at a time. After all, we can only live in today. If we have one foot stuck in yesterday and one foot stuck in tomorrow, we fail to acknowledge the here and now. We must remember that yesterday has passed, and tomorrow will come, so long as we just focus on today. It is natural for addicts to lack this perspective, as we tend to dwell on past mistakes and fixate on the future. But in doing so, we are wishing away the present. The present moment is most important in recovery, because it teaches us gratitude, patience, and perspective. With these ingredients, recovery is possible.

If things don't go the way I want them to one day, the next day is a fresh start. Promising myself to stay clean for the rest of my life can be daunting. Instead of biting off more than I can chew, I tell myself each day that I will not use that day. Taking this approach has made the thought of recovery more manageable. Of course, we all want to stay sober for the rest of our lives, but sometimes breaking things down into bitesize pieces makes them easier to digest. Rather than "for the rest of my life", remember, "one day at a time".

Chapter 6
How do I Deal with Relapse, Anyways?

You wake up in a cold sweat, your heart racing. You used last night. Your drug of choice, your usual rituals, your environment — all the same as before. Except it wasn't, because you're in bed and you were sleeping all night. Phew, that was a close one. It was just a dream...

Using dreams are quite common amongst addicts, and sometimes, they make us fear that we have relapsed. As a recovering addict, I am plagued with very intense and very frequent using dreams. While at first, I saw these as a relapse waiting to happen, now I see them as a gift. Not because I get to (somewhat) experience the pleasure of using again, but because it is not real. Using dreams can be very vivid in nature and thus very scary for the recovering addict. They may make us fear that we are not doing enough to recover or tempt us to use again. However, they also remind us of where we used to be and where we do not want to end up again. It is a sign of progress, rather than regress. When I had my first using dream, I went to my therapist very shaken up. He told me that I should be thankful for this dream — thankful that it was a dream (or a nightmare) and that it never really happened.

Dreams often reflect desires that we suppress during

the day. When we have using dreams, they can inform us to be more vigilant about managing these desires. For example, if I have a dream about using, I know that I need to be vigilant during the day in order not to use. These dreams make us more self-aware of our thoughts and emotions, and as a result, we are more equipped to deal with them in our everyday lives — without substances.

However, for some, relapse is not a dream but a reality. Relapse refers to using substances again after an abstinent period. It is estimated by the National Institute on Drug Abuse that forty to sixty percent of recovering addicts relapse at some point during their recovery. Yet, for alcohol and heroin users, this percentage nears ninety. Addicts may also relapse more than once, myself included. Just because you relapse does not mean your treatment has failed. Addiction is a brain disease that causes us to engage in compulsive substance use, even when we suffer negative repercussions as a result. The urge to relapse is ingrained in us, and sometimes, especially without proper treatment, we cannot fight it off.

There are many reasons why recovering individuals may relapse. It is all too easy to be a thirty or sixty-day wonder, then fall through the cracks back to your usual habits because, "Oh, it's just one drink," or "What harm will one do?" Or, it may be your environment causing you to justify using. "Everyone is having some, so I'll have some too," or "Hey, let's celebrate my success at work today." Reasons why recovering addicts relapse are manifold but may include the presence of triggers, lack of support after rehab, mental/physical pain, and young age.

First, an individual may be triggered to use again by a traumatic or stressful event in their life. As addicts, our learned way of coping with stress or trauma is by using to relieve the feelings associated with that stress or trauma. We use to forget, but never forget to use. Other, more simple triggers may also cause someone to use again. For example, passing by a bar they used to drink at or being in a social situation where drinks or drugs are available. When I came out of rehab, I decided to move apartments in order to avoid being triggered by my old using environment. However, removing triggers does not always solve the problem, nor is it always possible. What is key to learn here is how to handle your triggers, whether that's through meditation, mindfulness (see below), or a treatment program.

Another reason why addicts in recovery may resume using is due to lack of support after rehab or other treatment programs. The road to recovery does not end after treatment. It is a lifelong process. Thus, most addicts require continuous support following treatment, whether that means counseling, joining an anonymous addiction fellowship, or receiving aftercare treatment. Aftercare treatment includes prevention programs such as psychotherapy, the Twelve Steps, and sober living establishments, in order to extend care after completing treatment. Many people find these avenues useful in helping to maintain sobriety.

Next, physical or mental pain may prompt someone to relapse. Many people self-medicate as a result of physical or mental illnesses they suffer from. In order to cope with physical pain, such as chronic headaches, or mental pain, such as fatigue, stress, depression, or other psychiatric diagnoses, many people may resort to substance use. In my case, I self-medicated in order to balance out the symptoms of my bipolar disorder. When I was manic, downers were the answer; when I was depressive, uppers were. However, in recovery, these ailments will not cease to exist. We need to find more healthy, alternative solutions to these problems in order to cope.

Finally, some research has indicated that youth may play a role in relapse. When combined with psychiatric diagnoses, this risk is elevated. This is conceivable, given that psychiatric diagnoses often lead to self-medication. In particular, young patients may feel less equipped to deal with their psychiatric disorders than older, more experienced patients. Younger patients also have more time in which to relapse and may not be as educated about addiction and its consequences. Speaking for myself as a young addict, I tended to be very naïve when using substances. I figured, "I'm young, so what harm could they possibly do?" While I was lucky enough not to face any irreversible consequences of addiction (i.e., brain damage or death), some young people aren't so lucky.

Everything said, one method that studies suggest can help prevent relapse in recovering addicts is practicing mindfulness. Mindfulness is a technique used to bring people into the present moment. It teaches us how to be conscious and aware of our surroundings, while not being overwhelmed by them. Although I was skeptical of mindfulness when I was first introduced to it, there are many mindfulness activities that you can do depending on your likes and dislikes. It can be as simple as sitting in a silent room and noticing every sound happening around you, focusing on your breathing, or as complex as a listing game, like, "I'm packing a suitcase and I'm going to bring…" Whatever your preference is, mindfulness helps us remove ourselves from temptation by shifting our focus to the present moment.

However it comes about, relapse is not easy to come to terms with. After all, no one wants to feel like all of their hard work and dedication getting clean was put to waste. It can be extremely defeating to relapse, both for the addict and their loved ones. It can feel like the world is against you, and nothing you do is ever good enough. You may feel like a failure or a loser. You may believe you are not good enough to get clean for, because you'll just fall back into your old habits anyways. Although it's easier said than done, try not to be too down on yourself following a relapse. It will only make things worse and you may try to cope with the disappointment in yourself by using even more.

Following some of my earlier relapses, I figured there was no point trying to get clean. I would go a few weeks without substances, usually during family holidays, and end up racing my dealer back to my apartment to see who could get there first. Every time, I felt like I had failed myself. As a perfectionist, failure was not an option, so I figured, "Why even try to get clean any more? I'm better off giving in than trying and not being successful." The important thing to note though, is that failing lets us know that doing things a certain way won't work. We can learn from failure in order to be more successful in the future. And that's exactly what I did. I learned from each of my relapses, and eventually, something stuck. I no longer had to feel like a failure, because I was (and still am) a work in progress. I no longer had to feel like a loser, because I was winning myself back. Frankly speaking, relapse sucks, but it can serve an important purpose, if we choose to learn from it.

Rather than falling back into your old cycle, try to practice patience with yourself. Express gratitude that this was only a one-time thing. Learn from the experience and move on with your recovery. Don't get dragged down by your imperfection. Nobody is perfect, and nobody said recovery was easy. Bumps in the road are bound to happen. Rather than beat yourself up, try to stay positive and look ahead to the future. Just because you used today doesn't mean you have to tomorrow.

Relapse is difficult, but what matters is how you deal with it. After all, nobody's recovery is seamless. What you must realize is that your recovery is not defined by relapse. Your recovery is defined by how you handle its road bumps.

Chapter 7
Which Types of Treatment are Available Anyways?

Unfortunately, there is no magic pill to treat addiction. If there was, I don't think any of us would be in our position (or reading this book, for that matter). As addicts, getting treatment for our disease can be intimidating. You may not know where to start or what treatment is best for you. As previously discussed in other chapters, addiction therapy, inpatient/outpatient rehab, and anonymous addiction fellowships are all possibilities. This brief chapter will go into more depth about what each option entails and where to get started.

When I first realized I had a problem with drugs, I started by asking my doctor about addiction counseling in my area. She was able to refer me to a therapist that met all of my needs, who I saw once a week to try to work through my addiction. Lots of addiction counsellors are recovering addicts themselves and understand the underlying thoughts, emotions, and challenges that addicts face when still using and in recovery. In addiction therapy, you will explore the reasons for your using and your triggers, while learning methods to try to cope with your stressors in healthier ways. You will also celebrate your successes in recovery and will have someone to go to about addiction-related issues that you may not feel you can go to friends or family about. I decided to go to my addiction counsellor before most of my friends and family even knew I was suffering from addiction. I felt very alone facing my addiction at the time, and therapy really helped me feel supported. Even as a recovering addict, I still speak with my addiction counselor once a week in order to check in on my progress and discuss any challenges I may be facing, such as life events that make me want to start using again. Having someone to hold you accountable can be very helpful for battling addiction, though it may not be enough on its own for everybody.

It was my addiction therapist who referred me to rehab after seeing him for several months. Although my using had improved, it had not stopped, and he felt I needed more intensive treatment in order to get me into recovery. Rehab was a very frightening thought to me for a long time, because I felt that my using habits were not "bad enough" to justify the price and time spent in treatment. I was under the delusion that rehab was for "junkies", and I didn't fit that description. I felt like I would be an imposter attending rehab for my addiction, and that other people needed it more. I couldn't have been more wrong. In rehab, I attended lectures to learn more about the different facets of addiction, I went to group therapy twice a day to share experiences with other female addicts, I saw an individual therapist daily to speak about private issues in more depth, I began working through the Twelve Steps, and I was given assignments to apply what I was learning in treatment. Through all of these different modes of treatment in rehab, I gained invaluable skills to use in my recovery, and best of all, I learned more about myself. Learning about myself has proven extremely useful in overcoming my addiction, because I understand just how my brain works. Being more self-aware can help combat addiction, because you better understand your strengths, weaknesses, triggers, and barriers to recovery. Once you begin to truly understand yourself, you begin to recover.

However, I realize that inpatient rehab programs or addiction counseling may not be a financial possibility for everyone. Some inpatient rehabilitation centers do offer scholarships, and outpatient rehab also exists. These are typically cheaper and may also be funded by the government, depending on your income and where you live. While I don't have experience with any outpatient rehabilitation programs, the majority of drug treatment in Europe takes place in outpatient settings. The bottom line is that getting any kind of treatment for your addiction is better than none.

Another great option if you are strapped for cash is to find an anonymous addiction fellowship near you. Anonymous addiction fellowships are free and open to anyone struggling with addiction who wishes to get clean. You do not have to be in recovery yet to attend meetings. In meetings, members will discuss anything and everything related to addiction, as long as it is about themselves. One person speaks at a time, and everyone listens respectfully and without judgement. As a young addict, you may feel like your input is not as valuable as that of some of your older peers. However, sharing not only helps you make sense of your own addiction, but also helps other people in the fellowship make sense of their addiction. Remember, even older addicts were young once, too.

If you are an introvert like me, joining an anonymous addiction fellowship may not sound so appealing. However, you are not forced to speak at meetings if you do not want to, and newcomers are typically not expected to speak at their first meetings. Regardless if you decide to speak or not, joining an anonymous addiction fellowship is a great way to meet other addicts and relate to each other's' experiences. From my own experience, anonymous addiction fellowships are very welcoming, and their members want to help you in any way they can. As I've mentioned before, shared experience is what really helped me overcome my addiction. The solidarity felt by relating to other addicts is incredible — no matter how you find it — although, I acknowledge it may seem intimidating at first.

If you become a more regular member of an anonymous addiction fellowship, you may even be interested in finding a sponsor. A sponsor is an addict who has progressed in their recovery enough to share their experience with another addict trying to achieve or maintain sobriety. They have usually completed the Twelve Steps and regularly attend meetings with an anonymous addiction fellowship. While there are no formal rules as to how often sponsors should meet with their sponsees or exactly how the sponsor should help, they are generally there to offer additional support in times of need, help encourage their sponsees to regularly attend meetings and work through the Twelve Step program, and share their own personal experiences in recovery. If you are interested in getting a sponsor, all you have to do is ask. It is generally recommended that you find a sponsor who is the same gender as you and who has been clean for at least five years; however, as said before, there are no formal rules to sponsorship. Whether you decide to find a sponsor or just attend meetings, connecting with other addicts is a great way to feel supported in your journey towards sobriety.

As an addict, I know how frightening it is to admit you have a problem and seek help. While it may feel like a defeat, in reality it is a success! Admitting you have a problem with substances is the first step to achieving sobriety. Once you have accepted that you need help, there are resources available and waiting for you to take advantage of. All you have to do is have an open mind and want it for yourself.

Chapter 8
What is Life Like without Drugs, Anyways?

If you've ever heard the saying, "Once an addict, always an addict", you may be wondering why you need to stop using. If you'll always be an addict no matter what, what is the point? While it is true that addicts will always be addicts, even in recovery, this saying can be discouraging, given all the work that goes into recovery and living a healthy lifestyle post-active addiction. The saying fails to acknowledge that even though we are still addicts, we have changed our ways and are moving forward with our lives for the better. That said, I think what the saying is trying to convey is that addicts like us will always have to live with temptation. We cannot go to a party and use recreationally, like our peers may be able to. We cannot just have one drink and put down the pint glass. We must always be wary that we have a problem and do our best to stay away from substances for good. Once in recovery, it is all too easy to assume that we are "okay" again and to re-ignite the addiction we have healed from through all of our efforts to stay clean.

While temptations are something that addicts must learn to live with in recovery, they get easier to manage as time goes on. They become less and less frequent, and less and less intense. It is easier said than done; however, the longer you stay away from substances, the better you will feel and the stronger you will become. Temptations are not what defines life without drugs. What defines life without drugs is the improvement in the way you feel physically and mentally.

That said, it is not easy getting to that place. There is a lot of work to be done when getting clean. Many people use drugs in order to avoid problems they are facing in their everyday lives. I, for example, used in order to forget about my family situation, my mental health, academic stress, and my constant fear of never being good enough. However, when you begin your recovery process and stop using substances, all of these feelings and emotions you've been withholding come to the surface. At first, you may doubt that you even want to get clean if it means you have to tackle all of these things at once. However, once you overcome this initial stage of doubt, coping becomes easier.

When I first came out of rehab, I was lost as to how to cope with the overwhelming thoughts and emotions pouring out of me all of a sudden. I was doubting my educational path and my relationship. I didn't know what to do now that I couldn't conceal my feelings with a line, a joint, or a pill. My addiction therapist reassured me that all of these doubts and outpours of emotion were normal, because I was not hiding them with substances any more. In the end, once I began to get accustomed to this new way of life, I did end up transferring universities to study something new, and I stayed in my relationship, which I am still very satisfied with today. Believe it or not, recovery will actually add clarity to your life, rather than detract from it.

After reading all of this, you may be even more scared to stop using substances than you were before. Lots of work, temptation, and emotions may not sound so appealing. However, there is a silver lining. Through all of the struggles you may endure getting clean, you are one step closer to being the best version of yourself possible. You are one step closer to *you*.

Life without drugs can be daunting at first. However, the physical and mental effects of sobriety far outweigh the physical and mental effects of getting high. When you stop using, you start to feel yourself again. You become your own person without substances tying you down. Your academic/work life, family life, social life, and overall quality of life improve, not to mention your finances. The world takes a new shape, and you get to enjoy it again for the first time in a long time. Instead of chasing a high, you are chasing life.

First, your academic or work life will improve drastically when you dedicate yourself to sober living. You will regain the confidence, determination, motivation and ambition you may have lost as a result of using. All of the goals you once had that were tossed to the sidelines for substances will return, and you will be in the best place possible to achieve them. You will produce better work and receive better feedback. Most of all, whatever you do for school or work will be because of you. It will not be the substances achieving the results (or not). It will be your own hard work and commitment, and that is something to be proud of.

Your family life will also improve when you stop using substances. You no longer have to worry about being judged at family events or being frowned upon for your engagement with substances. You no longer have to feel alone in your battle with addiction, because family ties that were lost may be re-formed. You will be your best self for your family, and your relationships will benefit because of it.

Finally, your social life will blossom without substances by your side. In addition to being your best self for your family, you will be your best self for your friends and/or partner. They will no longer feel like they come second to substances, and you will benefit from their support as much as they will benefit from yours. You no longer have to decline invitations to social events because you are holed up in your room using or burden your friends or partner to babysit you while you are under the influence. Your relationships will become more genuine, more two-sided. You can give back as much as you get.

Overall, you will be amazed at how much better you feel every day. You will walk with your head held higher, with more pep in your step, with a new perspective on everything going on around you. Your physical health will not only improve, but so will your mental health. You no longer have to feel guilt and shame for using. You no longer have to feel alone in your struggle with addiction. When you open yourself up to the world, the world opens itself up to you.

Chapter 9
Why Should I Stop Using Now, Anyways?

When you're young, it is all too easy to justify using because you have so much time left to stop. We may say things like "I can stop when I want to," or "I'm still young, so it's fine." While it is true that you do have lots of time left to stop, the deeper you get into addiction, the harder it is going to be to come out of it. As young addicts, we often suffer from a sense of naiveté, thinking the consequences of addiction will never reach us. This is not the case. Being young does not make you immune to the dark side of addiction, nor does it make you immune to other illnesses like chicken pox or the flu. However, when we're young, our bodies are in better shape to cope with these illnesses, and the same can be said about addiction. Not in the sense that we are untouchable and nothing can harm us, but in the sense that we can catch the signs early and begin to address them, before the problem gets out of control.

I was lucky enough to have realized my addiction at the age of twenty-one, after using for one year. While this may not seem like a long time, addiction was my everyday routine. I would wake up, use substances, have breakfast, use some more, (maybe) go to class, come home, have lunch, and continue using until I went to sleep that night — sometimes at very late (or early) hours because I was using so much — only for the cycle to repeat again the next day. I didn't realize it at the time, but being dictated by substances is no way to live your life. All that time I was using, I was self-isolating in my room with little to no contact with the outside world, except for "emergency" trips to the grocery store when the munchies kicked in. I was lonely, I was struggling, and most of all, I was tired of substances being my everything. That's when I decided to get help.

Getting help does not mean your addiction will disappear overnight; however, it means you are on the right track towards recovery. It took me almost a year and a combination of addiction counselling, rehab, and joining an anonymous fellowship of other addicts to finally clean my slate of substances. Trust me, it is not easy, but getting sober is in your best interest.

While the effects of addiction may seem far from reality when you're young, the consequences mentioned in Chapter Three can affect any addict at any age. Health problems, relationship problems, financial problems, and problems at school/work will only worsen as your addiction goes on. That's why it is best to stop using sooner rather than later. When we stop, we can start repairing the damage done to all of these areas (where possible), and our lives will begin to come together again.

As young addicts, it is also easy to believe that our bodies are in good shape and can handle the adverse health effects that result from addiction. However, risks such as heart problems, brain damage, psychosis, and overdose can happen to anyone — even young people. Being tricked into thinking we are invincible is part of our disease and our youth. Using takes top priority despite these risks, because we are "healthy" or "young" or "different." The harsh reality is that's not true. We cannot see what is going on inside of our bodies, and you may not even know the toll substances have taken on it until it's too late. That's why it's important to stop using now.

The socio-economic consequences of your addiction will also worsen as your addiction worsens. Your school/work life, relationships, and financial state will only continue to fall apart. Your grades will continue to slip, your relationships will continue to break, and your finances will continue to disappear — until you decide you've had enough. When we stop using, all of these areas can begin to be mended, and you can begin to reach your full potential again. Until then, you must be prepared to handle whatever your addiction throws at you, and it's not always pretty. Again, that's why it is important to stop using now.

Once I stopped using substances, I noticed a significant difference in the way I felt physically and mentally. For the first time in a long time, my focus sharpened, my ambition returned and my overall mental health improved. I got an internship with a company I dreamed of working for, and I returned to my studies — this time online, in order to focus more on myself and my needs. None of this would have been possible without leaving substances behind. Take it from me, the only direction you can go after quitting substances is up.

Stopping now is not simple. It is probably the hardest thing you will ever do, and it may not be clear-cut. You may need treatment or relapse at some point throughout your recovery. At first, you may even miss your love affair with substances. This is all normal. However, deciding that you've had enough is a huge step in the right direction. As your sober time goes on, you will start to feel whole again. You will start to be you again.

It is easier said than done, but don't postpone your stop-date. Don't stop tomorrow, or after Johnny's birthday party, or after one last drink, joint, pill, line, or injection, because that may be too late. Stop *now*. Unfortunately, addiction can only lead us down three avenues: institutionalization, imprisonment, or death. If you haven't experienced any of these yet, don't go there. If you have, you probably don't want to go there again. Once you decide you're done, be done. Rid yourself of all the negativity substances have brought into your life, and seek out the positivity sobriety has to offer. Be the change you want to see in yourself. Getting clean is difficult, but it is necessary.

Being young complicates many areas of addiction. But it also simplifies some others. When we acknowledge our addiction early on, we have more time to enjoy a sober lifestyle. We have more time to get back what we may have lost. We have our entire lives ahead of us to be the best version of ourselves that we can possibly be — that's a gift. We are no longer in the grasp of addiction. Rather, we get a grasp on our addiction and begin to recover.

Chapter 10
Can Addicts be Friends in Recovery, Anyways?

Friendships are already difficult enough to manage as a young adult, without addiction getting in the way. However, as addicts, we must be extremely careful who we befriend. For many, substances provide the companionship they seek from others. For others, hanging out with the "wrong crowd" may encourage their use of substances even more. The bottom line is, substances are not our friends, and we must do everything we can to protect ourselves from their deceptive power. The friendships we do hold need to be honest, genuine, equal, and in our best interest.

The reason I bring up friendships is because many change throughout the course of addiction. You may make new (using) friends and discard old (non-using) ones, disconnect from friends entirely in order to use, or be excluded from social events because you are trying to get clean. Whatever shape your social life takes, it is sure to change as your behaviors change as well.

There are a few rules of thumb to follow when considering the intersection of friendship and addiction. First, staying friends with other addicts or heavy users when trying to get clean generally isn't a good idea.

Second, relationships of a sexual nature with people you meet in treatment of any kind is strongly discouraged. Finally, friendships with recovering addicts can be beneficial to both people involved, if the relationship is productive and non-using. The last thing you want is for your friends to derail the progress you are making in your recovery, or worsen your addiction.

First and foremost, it is best not to engage with other addicts when in recovery if they are not willing to change their ways. Although these individuals may seem like "friends", it is likely the friendship is based on using, rather than on a genuine, personal connection. These "friends" may help you justify using, be unable or unwilling to do normal activities sober, pressure you to use more, discourage you from getting help, or have no life apart from drugs. If this is the case, remaining friends while in recovery is a slippery slope to relapse. Even if these friends do not pressure you to use with them any more, the temptation to use and easy accessibility of substances is still there. You will always have someone to call in a moment of weakness to get your instant gratification.

Of course, cutting these ties is easier said than done. When I came out of treatment, I naively wanted to maintain all of my friendships, including those with my using friends. This was especially the case because I had grown distant from my non-using friends in the midst of my addiction. However, I did not find the support I needed in order to maintain my sobriety from these people. In the end, I had to make clear that the friendship wouldn't last if using was a requirement. Some of these people were able to accept that fact and adjust their behavior towards me, and some weren't. As a recovering addict who is hopefully working the Twelve Steps, this is something you will learn to make peace with. The world doesn't always work out the way you want it to; however, by following the Twelve Steps, you become more prepared to deal with undesirable outcomes. In recovery, you must remember that *you* come first. If your friendships are hindering your recovery rather than helping, it is best that you free yourself from their grasp.

Next, sexual relationships with people you meet in treatment, such as rehab or anonymous addiction fellowships, is a big no-no. Although you may feel comfortable doing so, especially given the very personal nature of these relationships, this is a dangerous game to play. If one partner relapses, it is much more likely that the second partner will too. In fact, most treatments have rules against relationships of a romantic or sexual nature exactly for this reason. For instance, when I was in rehab, relationships between opposite sexes were closely monitored in order to keep this risk under reigns. In addition, most anonymous addiction fellowships state in their mission that romantic relationships with newcomers are strongly discouraged in order to maintain the integrity of the program. If you are new to recovery, it is probably best that you are not involved in romantic relationships anyways, in order to focus on yourself. When I was in rehab, even communication with my non-using, long-term partner was discouraged, so that I could avoid distraction and fully focus on my treatment. No one is saying that you must end your relationship altogether if you enter treatment. In some cases, your partner may be very supportive and motivate you to get the help you need. However, it is generally agreed that you should not start a relationship with the individuals you meet in treatment, no matter how much they appear to be back on their feet. Again, the most important person in recovery is *you*, and anything or anyone that may deter you from progressing needs to stay out of the equation.

That said, friendships with other recovering addicts can be extremely beneficial to recovery. I spoke about this in Chapter Five, because this is what really helped my own recovery. The bonds you form with other people who understand your struggles can be very intimate. Finally, someone understands what you have been going through without you having to explain complicated backstories and reasoning you may not even understand yourself just yet. You both share an instant, common connection through your shared disease of addiction. This solidarity is truly something special and can help many recovering addicts understand themselves and their addictions better. However, when being friends with other recovering addicts that you meet in rehab, anonymous addiction fellowships, or other treatment programs, you must be wary of the risk that this friendship may not last if the other person relapses. When a friend stops attending meetings or turns back to their old ways, it can be difficult to process. We only want what is best for our friends, and knowing that they are struggling again can be very difficult to accept, especially when we may be at our best. It is okay to try to help these friends, but important that you do not sacrifice your own success or well-being in the process. You are at the center of your recovery, and you must always do what is best for *you*.

The bottom line is that friendships are beneficial, as long as they are a positive influence on our health and recovery. We should not feel pressured to use or be dissuaded from seeking help by our friends. Our friends should fully support our desire to get clean, whether that means getting us out of the house when we're going through a tough time or helping us find a treatment center in our area. Good friends provide support when we need it most. And, when we're the best version of ourselves, we are able to reciprocate. Friendships are give-and-take. When we are supported in our recovery, we begin to change for the better. When we are at our best, so too are our relationships.

Chapter 11
How do I Speak to my Loved Ones about Addiction, Anyways?

From my experience, people who have never suffered from addiction don't seem to want to talk about addiction. Whether that's because they're disinterested, uncomfortable approaching the topic, or unsure about what they can do to help, this makes it difficult to get the conversation rolling with your loved ones about your disease. When you open up about your own addiction, however, you may notice that this impassivity changes. After all, most people like to think that addiction will never touch their lives. When they realize that is does, their attitudes may shift, and hopefully, they will want to learn more about addiction alongside you.

That said, starting a conversation about addiction is not easy. If you're like me, coming clean about your addiction to friends and family may seem intimidating. You may not understand your addiction yourself just yet, and talking about it with others will only raise questions that you are not prepared to answer. When I first came out about my addiction, I was scared. Scared that I would be judged, condescended, or told that it was my fault. Most of all, I was scared that rejection from my loved ones would mean that I was still on my own to deal with my addiction — possibly even more alone, knowing that my friends and family didn't accept me. Besides, to them it probably seemed like I did this to myself. My family was a fan of the phrase, "You made your bed, so now you have to lay in it." In other words, I got myself addicted, so now I have to deal with the consequences.

Considering talking to your loved ones for the first time (or even second, or third) can be as daunting as admitting to yourself that you have a problem. The difference is, when you admit to yourself that you are an addict, you can take time to process it on your own terms. You may withdraw for a while, be in a state of denial, or use again to conceal the shame associated with recognizing you are an addict. In my mind, when I realized I was an addict, I decided I might as well live up to that description and use even more. Of course, this was not the right way to go about my acknowledgement, but perhaps the easiest at the time. When we admit to ourselves that we have a problem, we can recluse into ourselves and our addictions. When we talk to our loved ones about our addiction, we are opening ourselves up to harsh truths we may not be ready to face. We may not want to hear feedback like, "I always thought you had an addictive personality," or "I knew something was up with you." Or, we may not be ready to answer the question, "Where did I go wrong?" As addicts, we like to be in control of everything around us. Seeing our loved ones' reactions to the news of our addiction is something we cannot control or predict. We may be met with open arms or be scolded. We may realize that we have a support system or realize that we don't. This is extremely difficult, because in the unknown, there are many possibilities that we cannot control.

We already judge ourselves for being addicts, so feeling judged by our loved ones is the last thing we want. I was lucky enough to have gained the support of my family once I came clean about my addiction, but that doesn't mean it was easy. Seeing my loved ones' reactions to my announcement was extremely tough: lots of tears, questions, and sleepless nights. Nobody wants to see their loved ones hurt. Yet, the day I came clean was a big day for me. In admitting my addiction to my family, I also admitted my addiction to myself. I admitted that I needed help and that I couldn't do it alone.

If you are considering telling your loved ones about your addiction, the best advice I can give you is to be honest. Approach them in a private setting where public attention will not be drawn to whatever reaction your announcement may evoke. Make sure you share your news in a setting where both you and your loved one(s) will feel comfortable. Where possible, you may even want to tell more than one loved one at once, in order to avoid repeating the same difficult conversation, over and over again. While you do not want to make your addiction a public announcement, this may be a conversation that you only want to have once. Or, you may feel more comfortable approaching loved ones one by one. Everyone is different. Whatever you decide, take a deep breath and let it go. When we transfer the burden of our addiction onto other people, it doesn't feel like so much of a burden on us any more.

I chose to tell my family about my addiction after I

had been seeing my addiction therapist for quite some time. I thought that the fact I had taken action against my addiction would lighten the blow to my family and friends that I was an addict. In some ways I was right; in some ways I was wrong. Although they were proud of me for trying to tackle the issue with a therapist, it was still just as shocking for them to hear that I was suffering from addiction. None of my family had pegged me as an addict; although, they were aware of my bipolar disorder. What they didn't realize, however, was that my mental health was a significant contributor to my using.

Although most of my family was supportive of my bipolar disorder, some of them never fully understood my diagnosis. That's not to say that they weren't supportive, but they never truly understood the magnitude to which it affected my everyday life. The day I came clean about my addiction was the day all of that changed. I was met with a greater willingness to learn, readiness to listen, and desire to help from these family members. Had I not come clean about my addiction, none of them would have known the extent to which my mental health (and substance abuse) was interfering with my everyday functioning. In this way, opening up about my addiction was a positive experience.

That said, I was also confronted with some undeniable negatives. Although I felt less burdened, less alone, and more understood, I was also asked a lot of questions I did not necessarily want to answer. These questions were asked out of love and the desire to learn more about me and my addiction. However, they made me feel out of place, and I was not ready to speak so candidly about my addiction at that point. It is important to remember that most people do not know how to react to their loved ones being addicted, so rather than directly addressing the issue, they will resort to questions to feel more in control. If you are comfortable answering these questions, great. If you aren't, just save them for another time. Explain that certain questions aren't helpful or that you're not ready to speak about that topic just yet. Maybe you need more time to reflect before you're able to accurately answer some of these questions. Reinforce that when you are ready, you will come back to your loved ones. Until then, take your time to process the news that you just shared and the reactions received. Coming clean about your addiction can be a surreal experience, and it may have left you in a state of shock as great as that of your loved ones.

Although it's not easy, if you have a good relationship with friends or family, I would recommend telling them about your struggle with addiction. Keeping secrets is burdensome and makes us feel even more alone, when we're already at our lowest. Try not to worry about rejection. Your friends and family love you and want what is best for you. If they're not sure how to help you, or you're having trouble getting through to them, consider letting them read the next chapter of this book, *How can I Help an Addict, Anyways?* By providing a list of dos and don'ts, this chapter aims to help the loved ones of addicts navigate addiction. It is important to remember that addiction is not easy on anyone involved, including our loved ones. No one teaches us how to deal with these things in school. By having open conversations with our family and friends about addiction, we are educating others about what it means to be an addict. We are helping reduce the stigma that often accompanies our disease. Most of all, we are taking a massive step in our recovery, and that is something to be proud of.

Being scared to confront your family or friends about your addiction is normal. After all, it forces us to confront our addiction ourselves, which can be an uneasy process. However, it also may open up another outlet of support that you did not have before. When I was first considering telling my loved ones about my addiction, I hugely underestimated the leaps and bounds they would go through to help me. While that may not be everyone's situation, it is impossible to predict which response we will be confronted with. If it's not the one you were hoping for, remember that you are not alone. It may feel like it at the time, but other addicts are out there with similar struggles to you. Find them. Build a support network for yourself. Only together can we achieve recovery.

Chapter 12
How can I Help an Addict, Anyways?

If you know someone who is struggling with addiction, you may want to help but are not sure how. It can be confusing navigating addiction, both for the addict and for loved ones. Because there are so many misconceptions surrounding addiction (see Chapter One), many people do not understand what their loved ones are going through or what they can do to help. When considering supporting someone suffering from addiction, there are several dos and don'ts. While the list below is by no means exhaustive, its aim is to provide a framework as to where to start.

Do ask them how you can help. When you are feeling lost as to where to start, it may be best to simply ask what you can do to help your loved one. If they do not know, give them time to think about it and be ready to listen when they get back to you. If they do know, listen to what they are saying. To the best of your abilities, honor what they requested. Your loved one likely feels very alone in facing their addiction, and having someone support them along the way will mean a lot to them.

Do encourage them to get help. When you learn that someone you love is struggling with addiction, it can be a shock. I know this because my own family was very surprised when I came clean about my addiction. It can also be difficult to come to terms with. No one wants to imagine their loved one suffering. You may be very frightened or worried about them. You may feel sad. You may even feel angry. Everybody wants what is best for their loved ones, and when things do not go as planned, it is natural to react in these ways. However, rather than asking yourself what you did wrong, ask yourself what you can do right. Addiction is not anyone's fault, including the addict's, so blaming someone or something will not accomplish anything. What you can do is encourage them to get help. Whether this means holding an intervention or just having a conversation with your loved one, encourage them to see a therapist, attend meetings with an anonymous addiction fellowship, or go to rehab. Encourage them to talk to you about their addiction if and when they are comfortable. If they are not open to these ideas, give them time. Unfortunately, you cannot force someone to get treatment; they have to want it for themselves. The best you can do is point them in the right direction and be there for them when they are ready.

Do help them find treatment. When your loved one comes to you ready to get clean, help them find treatment that suits their needs. Even if they know they want help, many addicts lack the motivation to do this themselves. After all, the thought of setting off towards sobriety can be overwhelming for someone who has depended on substances for so long. Help them do their research, provide suggestions, and guide them towards an option that is right for them. However, it is important to remember that they must make the ultimate decision as to what is best for them. Just because your loved one may want to start with addiction counselling and not go straight to rehab, this doesn't mean they will never be ready for rehab. Any type of treatment is better than none and the fact that they are seeking help for the first time shows massive progress. Most types of treatment are interdependent anyways, so starting with one can lead your loved one down a path to another, if necessary.

Do invite them out when they're feeling down. By spending time with your loved one in a different environment, you can help distract them from the constant thought of using. Most addicts deal with hardship by using substances. This desire for substances is often non-stop and compulsive. Providing a healthy distraction from their troubles gives them a new outlet to enjoy rather than chemicals. Many addicts, including myself, hole themselves up in their room and self-isolate in order to use. Taking your loved one out can remind them that there is a world outside of substances, introducing them to new experiences.

Do send them a message to let them know you are thinking about them. If you are not able to spend time together in person, connecting to your loved one digitally can let them know that you care. Addicts often suffer from loneliness and self-isolation. They may avoid going out in favor of using or lose friendships as a result of their addiction. Simply sending them a message or giving them a call can help them feel more supported, even if from a distance. When I was in active addiction, I felt like nobody cared enough about me to know what was going on. After some sober-time, I've realized that this was not the case. However, substances often distort reality, and by making the extra effort to show your presence, you can make your loved one feel more fulfilled.

Do hold them accountable for their actions. This does not mean chastise them when they use after saying that they want to stop. This means set healthy boundaries that they can follow when they are around you. For example, if your loved one has a history of showing up to family gatherings under the influence, make clear that this is not appropriate under your roof. If your loved one pressures other family members to use with them, emphasize that there will be serious repercussions if they do this again. Most importantly, follow through. Setting boundaries may be difficult to do; however, addicts need them in order to recover. In fact, rehabilitation programs set many boundaries for the patients receiving treatment in their clinics. Patients must wake up, eat meals, and go to meetings at strict times. Setting expectations helps addicts stay on track towards recovery, even if they are not happy about it.

Do not enable your loved ones to engage in harmful behavior. This means do not give them money to buy substances, drive them to meet dealers, or use with them. This can be tough, as addicts are often very manipulative. However, by stopping sabotaging your loved one's recovery, you will be showing them tough love. Make clear that because you care about their wellbeing, you do not want to be part of anything that may harm them. Although they may be angry at first, in the long run, this will show them that you do not support their harmful behavior, even though you fully support them.

Do not interrogate your loved one about their addiction. There is nothing worse than being bombarded with questions when you come out as an addict. Instead, let your loved one come to you if and when they are ready to talk about it. When I first admitted my addiction to others, some members of my family responded by asking me about every little detail of my addiction, including what I use, how much, how often, how I use, who I use with, where I use, where I get my substances from, how they made me feel, and so on. Although this was a genuine attempt to understand my addiction, it made me feel awkward and judged. I was not ready to talk so frankly about my addiction and being expected to put me on the spot. You want to establish trust with your loved one, so do not push. This does not mean you cannot ask questions; however, limit them, and make sure the way they are being asked is in a productive way.

Do not judge or blame yourself or your loved one for their addiction. As stated before, addiction is not anyone's fault, nor is it a moral failing. It is not the result of bad choices; it is a disease that affects approximately thirty-one million people worldwide, according to the World Health Organization. Just because your loved one is suffering from an addiction does not change who they are on the inside. Everyone faces their own challenges in life and addiction happens to be theirs. Many addicts already feel enough guilt and shame as a result of their using habits, and it is not helpful if this guilt and shame is exacerbated by our loved ones.

Perhaps the best thing you can do if you have a loved

one struggling with addiction is educate yourself. Do your own research about addiction. Learn what it is, who it affects, and why. Learn the consequences of addiction and how you can help. If you are reading this book, that is already a good start. By learning about addiction on your own, you take pressure off of your loved one to explain it to you. They are already going through enough on their own and helping their friends and family to understand can be burdensome. What is most important is that your loved one focuses on themself, while trying to get the help they need. The more knowledgeable you are about their disease, the better you will be able to support them.

The list of dos and don'ts above is intended to help guide you through the process of supporting an addict in the most constructive way possible. While there is no right or wrong way to help, these suggestions are meant to provide a useful starting point from the perspective of an addict and the loved one of an addict (myself). If you have not read this entire book, I strongly encourage you to do so now. Each chapter is written from the perspective of a recovering addict and includes both factual and experiential information about addiction. Addiction is not one-size fits all. However, there are many common threads woven between addicts.

Conclusion

If you or somebody you know is struggling with addiction, you are not alone. You may not see other addicts around you, but that is because we are extremely good at hiding our addictions. Other addicts are out there, it just took me counselling, rehab, and becoming a member of an anonymous addiction fellowship to find them. Remember: Addiction does not discriminate. Addiction is a complex disease that can affect anyone, anywhere. It affects all ages, sexes, genders, races, religions, cultures, ethnicities, and socio-economic statuses. Millions are affected by addiction each year, including myself. As doctors and scientists conduct more research on addiction, we will continue to learn more about it. Hopefully this book has served as a good starting point to learn about addiction if you or somebody you know is struggling.

I hope this book especially reaches young addicts, who feel "left out of" addiction. Being young poses many challenges, and being a young addict is no exception. Although we may have different reference points than our older peers, keep in mind that addicts share many common threads. It may be trauma, neglect, guilt, or shame, but always remember that, despite being unique, we are one-of-a-kind. Together, we can combat addiction.

Together, we can dismantle the stigma surrounding our disease. Together, we can recover.

While recovery may seem far-fetched at first — especially in the midst of active addiction — it *is* possible. There are various resources available depending on your needs and abilities. For some people, addiction counselling may be sufficient. For others, like myself, it may take a long, personal journey through therapy, rehab, relapse, and membership to an anonymous addiction fellowship to begin to recover. Again, addiction is not one-size-fits-all. Everybody is different, but we share some similarities in our experiences as addicts. I hope this book has provided someone in need the reassurance and solidarity they needed to get through their addiction.

The most important thing is to never give up on yourself. You are worth getting clean for. Addiction is full of twists and turns, and I will be the first person to admit that it is a tumultuous journey. Nothing worth doing is ever easy. As you move through your journey towards sobriety, however, things will start to fall into place. You will start to see yourself and the world around you more clearly, and doors will open up that you never dreamt possible.

If you asked me when my addiction first started if I ever saw myself writing a book about addiction, I would have thought you were crazy. Of course not. I had no motivation, no ambition, and no desire to get clean. However, when I finally opened my mind up to new possibilities, new possibilities presented themselves to me. I have always been a writer, never really knowing which direction I wanted to take my passion. I remember tying together sheets of paper with yarn and calling it a book when I was a toddler. Now, here I am with a real book of my own. My dream finally came true, but it wouldn't have been possible had I continued using substances.

The moral of the story is that substances may seem like your friend, but in reality, they are your enemy. They prevent you from achieving what you can when you are clean. While you may think substances are helping you at first, things will eventually take a turn for the worst. Substances will no longer be your relief, but your restraint.

If you are reading this book, it is likely that you already want to change for the better. Don't lose sight of the change you want to be once you finish this page. Keep sight of your goal, and remember the only way to get there is by staying sober. You will be the best possible version of yourself once you are.

My name is Katelyn, and I am a recovering addict.

Additional Resources

For more information about Addiction:
- https://adf.org.au
- https://www.ccsa.ca
- https://www.drugabuse.gov
- https://www.samhsa.gov
- https://www.hazeldenbettyford.org/addiction/what
  -is-addiction

For Alcoholics:
- https://www.aa.org

For Addicts:
- https://www.na.org

For Loved Ones of Addicts:
- https://al-anon.org
- https://www.nar-anon.org
- https://www.farcanada.org
- https://www.hazeldenbettyford.org/addiction/help-
  for-families
- https://familyresourcectr.org
- https://adultchildren.org